Handling Grief

A Guide to Understanding and Coping with Loss

Dr. Ann B. Rhodes

Win 2 Publishing, LLC
Dr. Ann B. Rhodes, Owner
winllapastor921@yahoo.com
www.authorannbrhodes.com
www.facebook.com/annbrhodesauthor

Win 2 Publishing, LLC

Win 2 Publishing, LLC

Attn: Dr. Ann B. Rhodes

P.O. Box 156

Newnan, GA 30264

Email address: ann@win2publishing.com

Paperback ISBN: 978-1-7333222-9-4

Hardback 979-8-9876410-1-9

I dedicate this book to the memory of my beloved mother, Mrs. Alma Rhodes, whose presence and words of wisdom continue to inspire me and guide my steps. Your unconditional love, resilience, and unwavering support will always be kept inside of my heart. Thank you for being such a guiding light in my times of darkness and giving me the strength to cope with the depths of grief.

To my big brothers, both of you have been pillars of strength and sources of comfort. This dedication is for you. Your presence and listening ears have provided me solace in my times of sorrow. Your encouragement and friendship have illuminated my path.

To all those who have experienced the profound pain of loss and who have bravely embarked on their own journeys through grief, this book is dedicated to you. May its pages offer solace, understanding, and guidance as you navigate the complexities of mourning. May it serve as a reminder that you are not alone and that healing and hope are possible.

In remembrance of my beloved mother, Mrs. Alma Rhodes, and in honor of my cherished family members and friends, I offer this dedication. Your love, support, and memories have shaped this book and its purpose. It is my hope that <u>Handling Grief: A Guide to Understanding and Coping with Loss</u> serves as a beacon of light for all those who find themselves in the depths of sorrow.

Contents

Before you begin...

Grief is one of the most difficult things that a person can ever experience in their lifetime. I would like to thank you for joining me on this journey. To express that thanks, please accept a free copy of the Handling Grief Journal. Please scan the QR to let me know where to send your free gift.

This journal has been created to help you start the healing process in the challenges of grief. Grief contains many ups and downs, but make sure that you continue to trust in God during this challenging time. Handling Grief Downloadable Journal was created to help you express your feelings and to learn cope with the difficulty that comes along with grief. I hope that this journal will give you peace.

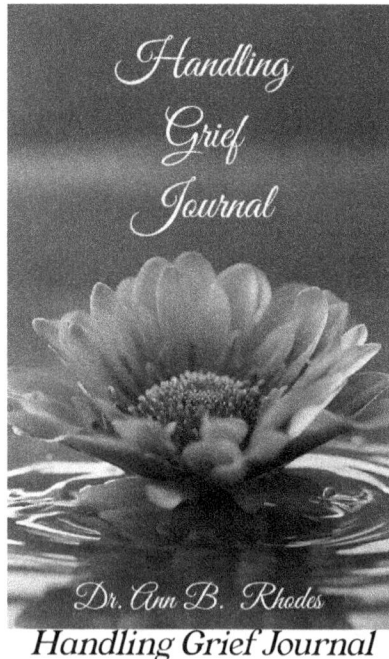

Handling Grief Journal

Chapter 1: Introduction to Grief

If you had asked me about grief before 2022, I really couldn't have given a good answer. I have had aunts, uncles, grandmothers, and grandfathers pass away, and I was sad over their deaths. I cried at their funerals and miss them even today. I still have a lot of memories about them. But my life completely changed on January 11, 2022, when my mother left her earthly home. When a person raised you, you always called them; you always checked on them; you went to see them leave this world; you have a better understanding on what grief is. My grandmother died in 1984, and my mother grieved every day and talked about missing her mother. My mother told me that one day I would understand what she was going through, and it is a pain that I would not wish for anyone to go through. Is grief something you get over? No, it is not. You can only learn to accept it and adjust to a new norm. Is it difficult to adjust? Yes, it is. I can only make it through by knowing my mother is watching over me daily and I will apply what she taught me throughout the years. I have a better understanding of all the things she told me years ago. I have pictures and videos to look at that I value more than ever.

Section 1: What is grief?

As I reflect on answering the question about defining what grief is, my typical answer would be that it is a natural response of how we act when a loss takes place. Grief comes with emotional, physical, and cognitive responses of losing someone or something that someone cares a great deal about. When I think of grief, I automatically associate it with the death of a loved one, but a sense of grief can also be experienced with a relationship ending, job loss, health decline, or a loss of a big dream or expectation.

Grief is one of the strongest influences on a person. It could change their entire life. Grief can manifest itself as sadness, anger, guilt, regret, and confusion. The time needed to grieve varies from person to person. It is influenced by the type of loss, how the person copes with the loss, and the type of support that is around them.

A person never stops grieving. You just learn how to live with significant change. Grief can take place in different stages and time periods. It is often followed by periods or stages that include sadness, anger, bitterness, and the acceptance of grief. Grief can affect a person physically. A person's appetite, sleeping patterns, and even energy level can change. The cognitive function of a person can also be impacted by grief. This can lead to a person having difficulty with concentration, memory, and decision-making. The way a person is grieving will often change socializing habits.

When the word grief comes to mind, pain and sorrow follow immediately. Grief is a true expression of the love, attachment, and how significant a person was to the person who has suffered a loss. It's a natural process to honor the person whom you have had a connection to and process the loss of a loved one. It is also a way to continue with the absence of a loved one. A person may ask, is there a certain way to grieve? The answer is that there is no right or wrong way to grieve. Everyone's journey in grief is different based on their personality, culture, beliefs, and support system. By understanding grief, it will allow compassion, empathy, and support for oneself and others who are encountering the difficult task of dealing with grief.

Section 2: Types of grief

When the thought came to my mind about writing a book on grief, I had to google types of grief. As I experienced the grieving process, it is important to note that there are two types of grief which include anticipatory and disenfranchised grief. A variety of different experiences may trigger these types of grief. Anticipatory grief begins before the actual loss of a loved one occurs. This source of grief begins when someone expects the death or loss of a loved one because of a terminal illness, older age, or a long-term condition. This type of grief prepares a person for a loss, so the grieving process starts early. With anticipatory grief, an individual can make reflections, and connections, and sometimes talk to the person who is dying in order to get closure and peace before the loss of a loved one occurs.

Disenfranchised grief is a type of grief that is not openly acknowledged or even recognized by most people. Examples of this type of grief include the death of a pet or the loss of a non-martial relationship. Many people feel a type of isolation. They are often misunderstood during the healing process. It really doesn't matter what type of grief a person is going through, people should offer support and understanding to anyone who is experiencing it.

Section 3: Stages of grief

Even though grieving is a natural part of loss, it is a complex way a person deals with a wide variety of emotions, thoughts, and behaviors. People typically go through five stages of grieving which include: denial, anger, bargaining, depression, and acceptance. It is important to remember that everyone goes through the grieving process differently. Everyone will not experience every stage and the stages of grief will hit everyone in a different order.

Denial is one of the first stages in the grieving process because people have a difficult time accepting the idea of any kind of loss. My mother was a strong, courageous woman who taught me many life lessons about how to tackle this world on my own. There are so many days that it doesn't seem real and yes, I am still in the denial stage. I still leave a place at the dining room table where she always sat with her apron that marks her space. No one should dare sit in my mother's spot because I will visibly get upset and snap at anyone who tries to take her spot at the dining room table. Some days hit me harder than others because I simply question why do I have to experience a pain that goes so deep? My mother and I were like inseparable twins. Where you saw one, you would see the other. When I go to my mother's house, I expect her to be sitting in the living room in her recliner chair with the television on, watching the Price is Right, Matlock, QVC, HSN, the news, or the Young and the Restless. Now, all I get is an empty living room where I sit, stare, and reflect on the memories that my mother left me. There are so many times that my brothers and I reflect on some things that my mother always told us and that "my mother was always right."

Sometimes I feel a sense of anger that my mother is gone. I often sit in front of a picture of my mother crying, asking, "Mommy, why did you have to leave me? Nothing is the same without you here on earth." It took me several months after my mother's death before I could even go to the grocery store alone. Each time I would step foot into a grocery store, I would cry. Why? Every Saturday morning, I would head to my mother's house and we would go grocery shopping. We would go to Food Depot and Piggly Wiggly to get groceries; we would go to Wal-Mart to pick up a couple of items and head home. I remember backing up the car and getting the groceries out of the car and handing them to my mother on the back steps of the deck porch. We had a deep freezer. All of the groceries we bought we put at the bottom and then put all the food that we hadn't cooked yet on top. We would keep our freezer full so we always had plenty of food to eat. I still think about those trips on Saturday mornings because now I have to take on the challenge of going grocery shopping alone. I talk to God often, trying to put things in perspective, but I still don't understand why.

One thing that many people don't realize is that I went through a deep depression. I cried for several weeks because my daily routine included going straight to my mother's house after I got off of work. I never missed a day. Anytime it was break time at work, I would always call my mother. It was a big transition not to do that anymore. At the time of my mother's death, I was enrolled in an online college class. This class started on a Monday and my mother passed away on Tuesday. My initial thought was to drop out of the class, but after a conversation with my brothers, they said, "Mommy would want you to finish." So, I contacted my professor and told her about my situation, and asked for an extension on my assignments. My extension was granted, and I continued to work full-time while taking my college class. This class was the last class I needed to finish my degree. It was the best decision that I made to continue with the class because it helped to take my mind off of the situation. I could stay busy so that I would not go into a really deep depression. My mindset changed because now I was going to finish this class and graduate in "my mother's honor". I had something that I was going to work toward to make my mother proud. I look at her picture every morning and throughout the day. I had to do something in order to function.

Although I know my mother was gone in the physical realm, I can still feel her presence in the spiritual realm. It is difficult for me to accept the fact that she is truly gone and she is not coming back. I often remember several conversations that she had with my brothers and me that I never wanted to hear. She always told her children "This is not your home. We did not come here to stay." I can definitely say that she was right. We never know the day or the hour that God will call us home. We always need to be prepared and ready. You should always have a good relationship with God. Do I accept the fact that my mother is gone? I don't. Sometimes I am waiting to find her sitting in the living room in her favorite chair at her house. I still have her phone and other things that I will always cherish and take care of for as long as I shall live. If a parent that you are close to leaves you, then the sense of emptiness never goes away. You will always feel a sense of aloneness.

Bargaining is another stage of the grieving process. During this stage of grieving, a person may attempt to negotiate with a higher power to reverse or ease the pain. I remember when a friend lost a family member she was very close to. She would always visit a place where she would always go with them on a regular basis. She would look up to the sky attempting to negotiate with a higher power to reverse the agony and pain, hoping that this was all a dream. She desperately wanted a second chance. This stage of grief was an example of how a person can release anguish in an attempt to find solace amid the unimaginable pain. Grief can drive individuals to seek reprieve from a higher power when confronted with circumstances beyond their control. It is a way of trying to control the situation. Depression often comes with feelings of emptiness, sadness, and a sense of loss.

Although bargaining is a stage of grieving, one of the most difficult stages in grieving is the stage of acceptance. Acceptance is not about forgetting the person, but it is about coping with the loss of a loved one. I have learned to accept "my new normal" in life. I will always carry my mother's memories and traditions.

It is important to remember that everyone handles grief in different ways. The grieving process is different for every person. The period of grief for an intense person can last for a shorter time. But some people grieve for an extended period of time.

With the grieving process, it is important to remember that people need to be gentle and get all the support that they need from others. Often, people have to lean on their family and friends, join support groups, or get help from a skilled counselor or therapist. Self-care, patience, and allowing oneself to experience and express any emotions are important during the grieving process.

In short, grieving includes emotions, stages, and different experiences. It is a process that includes adaptation and healing as a person finally accepts the loss of a loved one and moves forward in order to honor the special person or animal that they have lost.

Section 4: Identifying some myths and grief

There are several myths and misconceptions that people have about the grieving process. These beliefs impact the process. In order to have a better understanding of the myths and misconceptions, I am going to give you information that will include both a misconception and a fact.

Misconception: Grief has a specific time period or timeline.

Fact: No one ever gets over the grieving process. I remember in my mother's lifetime; she grieved for her mother from 1984 until her death in 2022. So I know for a fact that grieving doesn't have a timeline. People need to remember there is no "right" or "wrong way" to grieve.

Misconception: Grief is something that you need to get over.

Fact: Grief is a natural process that occurs when a loss happens. Everyone deals with grief differently. It takes time for each person. The healing process is a gradual and ongoing process because people have to adjust to the new reality of living without a loved one. A person must learn how to move forward with their life.

Misconception: If you show people you are grieving, then you are a weak person.

Fact: Let's remember that grieving is a healthy process, and it is a necessary part of life. It takes courage in order for people to show their emotions. Denying grief can only lead to emotional and health issues.

Misconception: Grief will only affect your emotions.

Fact: Grief can affect people emotionally, physically, cognitively, and spiritually. It can make people physically sick, mess with a person's cognitive process, and cause a person to question what they believe in. It is important to understand grief from a holistic point of view so people can address the various components of grief.

Misconception: In time, feelings of grief will heal.

Fact: There is no amount of time that will heal grief. Time can bring healing and perspective; time will not resolve grief. The actions of healing and change occur when you have support and coping mechanisms to handle your grief.

Misconception: Grief will end after the funeral or memorial service.

Fact: More than likely, grief is higher immediately after losing a loved one. It is an ongoing process of mourning because a person has to adjust to living without someone or something that they may have lost.

Misconception: People should handle grief alone and be strong.

Fact: During the period of grief, people need all the support that they can get. Grief is overwhelming and people need support from loved ones, support groups, or professional counselors. If a person is asking for help, that is a sign of strength, not weakness. Talking to other people who have experienced the same grief as you have can provide you with sound advice and understanding.

Misconception: Everyone grieves the same.

Fact: Grief is different for everyone. No two people will grieve the same. Factors that influence grief include culture, personality, and the type of loss the person has experienced. You can't compare one person's grief to another person's grief. Everyone is different and reacts to things differently.

By recognizing the myths and facts about the grieving process, a person can better understand how to be compassionate and supportive of someone experiencing grief. It is important to understand the complexity of grief in order to have empathy, understanding, and support for people who are going through the challenge of loss and the healing process.

Chapter 2: Understanding Loss

Can you ever understand the loss of a loved one? No, I can't. I can only think back to things that my mother would say and try to explain to my brothers. I didn't understand it then, but now I have a clear understanding. My mother always said, "This is not our home. We didn't come here to stay." I must say that is so true. I never liked my mother talking like that, but she was preparing her children years ago for the moment she was going to leave us and go back to Jesus. She always told us, "Do not be afraid. We are not better than anyone else." Just reflecting back on those very words, I can say that my mother was always right. I can only dream of being the woman that she was and carrying out all of her wishes.

Section 1: The types of loss

Grief can be triggered by a variety of losses. It doesn't have to be a loss of a loved one. Often, people associate grief with the death of a loved one, but it is important to understand the different losses that can occur in a person's life that may make them grieve. Examples of significant types of grief include:

Death

If you lose someone that you are close to then, that is an automatic trigger for grief. This includes a family member, a close friend, or a pet that can lead to sadness and a pure emptiness inside. Grief causes a person to go through a change period of mourning the physical loss of the person, making a life change without the person, and processing the situation of the loss emotionally. I recently saw a person whom I went to high school with, but he was much older than me. I knew his family very well, but the family grew apart after his mother and father's death. Parents are the glue that keeps the family together, but when they leave this world some families fall apart. I saw him from a distance at the side of the road in a wheelchair with a sign up that said he was in need of money. One of his legs had been amputated. My heart truly went out to him because he was a person who I knew and when I saw him last year, he had a job and seemed fine. It's amazing how things can change in a blink of an eye.

Divorce or Relationship Breakdown

When a relationship ends, such as a divorce or a long-term relationship, grief can occur. A person's heart is shattered because of the dreams, aspirations, and future plans have been interrupted and have come to a complete stop. A lot of emotions are involved in a breakup because one has to redefine their own identity and navigate the complexity of being a co-parent with an ex-partner or maintaining other connections with the person.

Job Loss or Career Change

Any time a person loses a job or has a change in their career, they will experience grief. People can feel insecure with identity loss; and financial strain. Individuals could mourn routines, social connections, and a sense of purpose associated with their work. A job loss involves a lot of emotions, seeking new employment opportunities, and adapting to a changed professional landscape. I remember when I was teaching at my first school for thirteen years. Human Resources moved me to a different school before the next school year began. I was hurt because I had been at my first school for so many years. I did not want to move, but my contract said, "I work for the county and not the school." I lost the relationships I had with coworkers, parents, and students. It was definitely a hard loss.

Health Decline or Chronic Illness

Anytime a person has a change in a health condition or a chronic illness, it can cause grief. Sometimes people have a loss in the way their body functions in order to complete certain tasks, including not being as independent as they once were. When people have a new limitation or a lifestyle change, then it will impact them emotionally as well as impact their relationships with other people.

Miscarriage or Pregnancy Loss

Pregnancy loss can present grief. Individuals and couples are often devastated because they will think about what type of future they could have had with their unborn child. Grieving can include a source of various emotions, physical and hormonal changes, support from healthcare professionals, and support groups.

Loss of Home or Relocation

If someone needs to move because of a natural disaster, financial difficulty, or any type of forced migration that could be a cause of grief. When people have adjusted to a certain type of environment or made connections with people, then it is a huge loss. Stability is important to a person. Now a person must adjust to a new surrounding and process the emotional impact of being displaced from their home. They must now transition to a new place.

These are just a few examples of a loss that a person can experience. Everyone must understand that the people grieve differently. We must provide support for one another during the grieving process.

Section 2: The impact loss has on our lives

Anytime someone experiences a sense of loss, it can be profound and life-changing. It doesn't matter if it involves a loss of a loved one, the end of a relationship, or a loss of job, it can heavily impact a person's life. The impact of a loss can be shown in people in a variety of ways.

Emotional impact

When a person experiences a loss, it will include a variety of emotions. Common emotional responses to grief include sadness, anger, guilt, confusion, and even relief. These emotions can fluctuate over time and be quite overwhelming. A feeling of emptiness and sadness can be felt for an extended period. Grief can affect how a person functions daily, their relationships with others, and their overall well-being.

Physical impact

Loss can have an effect on people physically, also. People can have issues physically that could include fatigue, changes in appetite, fatigue, fluctuation in weight, headache, and gastrointestinal issues. The stress and emotional toll of loss can impact the body's physiological functioning and cause various physical symptoms.

Cognitive impact

Grief can impact a person's cognitive functioning a great deal. Concentration, memory, and decision-making can run into cognitive overload. The processing of grief requires mental and emotional energy, which can temporarily impact cognitive functioning. This cognitive fog or "grief brain" can make it challenging to focus on tasks, solve problems, or retain information.

Social impact

Loss can have a profound impact on an individual's social life and relationships. Grieving individuals may feel a sense of loneliness as they may struggle to relate to others who have not experienced a similar loss. Social interactions may be strained, as individuals navigate their own grief while also trying to support others or maintain their pre-existing roles and responsibilities. Individuals may need to establish new support networks or find solace in support groups with others who have gone through similar experiences.

Identity and meaning

Loss can deeply challenge an individual's sense of self and purpose. Significant losses can disrupt one's identity, life trajectory, and personal beliefs. Individuals may question their own values and life goals and may reevaluate their place in the world. The search for meaning and purpose in the aftermath of loss can be a profound and ongoing process. I often question my place and purpose in life at this very point. Some days are better than others, but I still try to continue to move forward.

Spiritual and existential impact

For many individuals, loss raises profound existential questions and may lead to a reevaluation of spiritual or philosophical beliefs. The search for understanding, comfort, and a sense of connection to something larger than oneself can become more pronounced during times of loss. Individuals may seek solace in their spirituality, engage in philosophical reflections, or explore existential questions related to the nature of life and death. I have several questions about the life which include: How much does a person watch over you? Are they still aware of what is going on in this world? Will they actually rise from the dead one day? Can the spirit of the person talk or show you signs of something?

Section 3: Factors that can influence grief

Grief is a difficult experience and can be influenced by various factors that can complicate the healing process. Understanding these factors is important for individuals dealing with the journey of grief. In this section, we will explore some of the common elements that can complicate grief, shedding light on their impact and offering insights for those grappling with their effects.

Traumatic Loss

Grief can become more complicated when the loss is traumatic. Traumatic losses, such as sudden deaths, accidents, or acts of violence, can leave individuals with intense feelings of shock, disbelief, and profound emotional distress. The sudden and unexpected nature of these losses can make it challenging for individuals to process their grief and integrate the reality of the loss into their lives.

Complicated Relationships

The dynamics of a relationship with the deceased can also complicate the grieving process. Conflicting emotions, unresolved conflicts, or strained relationships can leave individuals with complicated feelings of guilt, anger, or unresolved issues. Losing a loved one with whom the relationship was difficult or ambivalent can create a unique set of challenges in the grieving process.

Previous Losses or Trauma

Past experiences of loss or trauma can significantly impact how an individual grieves in the present. Unresolved grief from previous losses or traumatic experiences can resurface and intertwine with the current grief, amplifying its intensity. It is important to recognize and address these underlying layers of grief to facilitate healing and prevent further complications.

Lack of Support

Grieving in an unsupportive or invalidating environment can complicate the healing process. When individuals are not met with understanding, empathy, or validation for their grief, they may struggle to express their emotions or seek the support they need. The absence of a supportive network or encountering dismissive attitudes can impede the grieving process and prolong the pain.

Difficult Circumstances Surrounding the Loss:

Certain circumstances surrounding the loss can complicate the grief experience. For example, legal battles, financial strains, or other practical challenges can add additional layers of stress and uncertainty to the grieving process. External factors that disrupt the mourning rituals or the inability to honor the deceased can also complicate the healing journey.

Cultural or Religious Factors

Cultural and religious beliefs, rituals, and expectations can influence how grief is expressed and experienced. Conflicting expectations of cultural or religious practices can create additional layers of complexity in the grieving process. Coping with these dynamics while honoring personal beliefs and finding meaning in loss can be a challenging endeavor.

Co-occurring Mental Health Conditions

Grief can coincide with pre-existing mental health conditions or trigger the onset of new ones. Conditions such as depression, anxiety, post-traumatic stress disorder (PTSD), or substance abuse can complicate the grieving process and require specialized support and treatment.

It is important to recognize that complications in grief are not indicative of weakness or failure. They are a natural response to unique circumstances and individual differences. Seeking support from compassionate professionals, engaging in self-care practices, and allowing oneself the time and space to heal are vital steps in navigating the complexities of grief. By acknowledging and understanding these factors, individuals can find resilience and hope as they continue on their journey of healing.

Chapter 3: Coping with Grief

I am not going to lie. Coping with grief is probably one of the most difficult things that you will encounter in your life. The first couple of months of my mother's death were rough. All of my daily routines were gone. I couldn't call her phone, because I knew that she couldn't answer. When I'd go to her house, I would only go into empty space. Crying is something I did everyday for several months. Even the slightest thing that involved "mom" made me emotional. Then one day, it hit me. My mother would want me to be strong. Even in her absence, she still has a way to guide me.

Section 1: How to handle self-care through grief

Self-care plays a crucial role in navigating the challenging roles of grief. When we experience loss, our emotional, physical, and spiritual well-being can be deeply impacted. It is during these times of intense sorrow and upheaval that practicing self-care becomes even more essential. In this section, we will explore various strategies and approaches to self-care that can support individuals in their healing journey.

Honor Your Emotions

Allow yourself to feel and express your emotions without judgment. Grief encompasses a wide range of emotions, from sadness and anger to guilt and confusion. Give yourself permission to experience these emotions and find healthy ways to express them, for example, through journaling, talking to a trusted friend, or engaging in creative outlets like art or music. A day after my mother died, I wrote a poem titled, "My Mother, my Angel."I decided to read it at her funeral. It was the best way to give my final tribute to my mother. I also placed each book that I had written in the casket with her. I hope that she will remember how much I loved her and will miss her.

Get Your Rest and Sleep

Grief takes a toll on both the mind and body, and adequate rest and sleep are important for healing. Make self-care a priority by establishing healthy sleep habits and creating a soothing bedtime routine. Practice relaxation techniques such as deep breathing, meditation, or gentle yoga to promote restful sleep and overall well-being.

Nourish Your Body

Grief can disrupt appetite and eating patterns, but it's important to nourish your body with healthy foods. Focus on consuming a balanced diet that includes fruits, vegetables, lean proteins, and whole grains. Stay hydrated and try to limit excessive caffeine or alcohol intake, as they can exacerbate feelings of anxiety or restlessness.

Engage in Gentle Exercise

Physical activity can be a powerful tool for managing grief. Engage in gentle exercises such as walking, swimming, or yoga to release tension, boost mood, and increase energy levels. Listen to your body's needs and find activities that feel nurturing and supportive.

Seek Support

Surround yourself with a supportive network of friends, family, or a grief support group. Reach out for help when needed and lean on others who can provide a compassionate ear or a comforting presence. Share your feelings and experiences, and remember that you do not have to navigate grief alone. I was able to lean on friends who knew exactly what I was going through. I remember when a close friend lost her mother years ago, I was there for her. When she got the news of my mother, she was there for me too. It truly meant a lot to have someone to talk to who understood the pain that I was going through.

Establish Rituals

Rituals can provide a sense of structure, comfort, and meaning during times of grief. Create personal rituals that honor your loved one or the loss you are experiencing. This could be lighting a candle, visiting a special place, writing in a journal, or engaging in a mindful activity that holds significance for you. One particular thing that my mother did was cook for the family every Sunday. In fact, she would begin cooking on a Saturday and finished up cooking on Sunday morning. I am proud to say that I have continued that tradition. My mother always told her children, "If something ever happens to me, I want y'all to come back to the home house." So for each holiday, we eat at my mother's house.

Practice Self-Compassion

Be kind and gentle with yourself throughout the grieving process. Acknowledge that grief takes time, and that healing is not linear. Treat yourself with compassion, embracing your own unique journey of grief. Allow yourself to rest when needed, set boundaries, and grant yourself permission to prioritize your own well-being.

Engage in Activities that Bring Joy

While grief is accompanied by pain, it is also important to find moments of joy and pleasure amidst the sorrow. Engage in activities that bring you joy, whether it's spending time in nature, reading a favorite book, listening to uplifting music, or pursuing a hobby. Allow yourself to experience moments of respite and find solace in the things that bring you comfort and happiness. I try to go out to eat with friends and get my nails and toes done once a month.

Remember that self-care is not selfish; it is an act of self-preservation and healing. Your well-being is importa nt. You are better equipped to take on the challenges of grief and find moments of peace and renewal. Take small steps each day to care for yourself; and know that you are worthy of the love, compassion, and care you extend to others.

Section 2: Identifying strategies to manage grief

As stated earlier, grief is complex. It can lead to a series of symptoms and challenges. It is important to have strategies in place to manage these symptoms effectively, as they can significantly impact our daily lives. In this section, I will explore practical and holistic approaches to address common grief symptoms and help individuals find relief and healing.

Addressing Emotional Symptoms:

Expressive Writing

Writing can be a powerful outlet for processing emotions. Encourage individuals to keep a grief journal where they can freely express their thoughts, feelings, and memories related to their loss. This act of writing allows for reflection, emotional release, and gaining insights into their grief journey. As I have already stated in this book, I wrote a poem the day after my mother passed away and read it at her funeral. It was my way of expressing my feelings to others at that event.

Seek Counseling or Therapy

Professional support can provide a safe and compassionate space to explore and navigate the complex emotions associated with grief. Therapists or grief counselors can offer guidance, coping strategies, and validation, helping individuals work through their emotions in a supportive environment. I did not seek professional help for grief, but the thought crossed my mind several times.

Practice Mindfulness and Meditation

Mindfulness techniques, such as deep breathing, meditation, or guided imagery, can help individuals cultivate present-moment awareness and reduce stress. These practices promote relaxation, emotional regulation, and a sense of grounding amidst the tumult of grief.

Managing Physical Symptoms

Prioritize Rest and Sleep

Grief can often disrupt sleep patterns, leading to fatigue and exhaustion. It is vital to establish a consistent sleep routine, create a soothing bedtime environment, and practice relaxation techniques before bed to have good sleep.

Engage in Gentle Exercise

Exercising helps with physical symptoms associated with grief which include tension, restlessness, and lethargy. Walking, yoga, and stretching, are exercises that improve a person's mood, boost energy levels, and help a person's overall well-being. Regular physical activity can helps alleviate physical symptoms associated with grief, such as tension, restlessness, and lethargy. Encourage individuals to engage in gentle exercises like walking, yoga, or stretching, which can improve mood, boost energy levels, and promote overall well-being.

Practice Relaxation Techniques

Deep breathing exercises, progressive muscle relaxation, or engaging in calming activities like taking a warm bath or listening to soothing music can help reduce muscle tension, ease anxiety, and promote relaxation.

Coping with Cognitive Symptoms

Practice Self-Compassion

Grief often brings about self-critical thoughts and feelings of guilt. We must encourage ourselves to practice self-compassion by offering kindness, understanding, and acceptance. We have to be reminded that grief is a natural response to loss, and it is okay to feel and process their emotions at their own pace. I often ask myself, could I have done more? That will forever and always be in the back of my mind.

Seek Mental Stimulation

Engage in mentally stimulating activities, such as reading, puzzles, or learning a new skill. These activities can help redirect focus and promote cognitive well-being. They provide purpose, improve cognitive function, and offer a temporary respite from the intensity of grief. It is important to stay busy, but understand that you can not ignore grief. You have to have a sense of peace that you did all that you could do.

Use Memory Triggers

I have several objects that serve as memories of my mother. I have her purse, jewelry, clothes, photographs, dishes, and much more that hold a strong sentimental value. These memory triggers can provide comfort, foster a sense of connection, and keep cherished memories alive. I look at my mother's picture every day. On occasion, I look at videos of family times of her birthday, Mother's Day, Christmas, and Valentine's Day. It can be emotional to watch those videos so I watch them during the times that I am strong and when I miss my mother tremendously.

Finding Social Support

Join Support Groups

Connecting with others who have experienced similar losses can be immensely beneficial. Support groups provide a safe space to share experiences, receive validation, and gain insights from others who are on a similar grief journey. No one knows what you are experiencing unless they have encountered the same situation. As I stated before, a close friend of mine who lost her mother a couple of years ago was there for me when I lost mine. Just to talk to someone and cry with someone who truly understood what I was going through meant a lot and really helped me through the grieving process. There were people who told me that if I just needed to pick up the phone and cry, I could call them. I had some coworkers who had encountered my experience that I could fall back on at work. I definitely had a strong support system.

Seek Companionship

Engaging in activities with friends, family members, or trusted individuals who provide comfort and companionship is important. Spending time with loved ones who understand and support the grieving process can help alleviate feelings of isolation and foster a sense of belonging.

A coworker of mine who lost her mother years ago enjoys going to Family Feud. The studio is in south Fulton County. She invited me to go to be in the audience with her. I told my brother about it, so he came along with some other coworkers and friends. I had so much fun that a couple of weeks later, I went back with both of my brothers. It's always good to get together and just have fun with family and friends.

Seek Professional Support

If social support is limited, or if individuals feel the need for additional guidance, professional grief counselors or therapists can provide invaluable support and guidance throughout the grieving process.

Managing grief symptoms is a personal and evolving process. It is essential to find strategies that resonate with each individual's unique needs and preferences. By addressing emotional, physical, cognitive, and social symptoms, individuals can develop a comprehensive toolkit for managing grief and finding renewed hope and healing.

Section 3: The role and purpose of support networks

Support networks play a vital role in the journey of grief, providing comfort, understanding, and guidance to individuals navigating the complex emotions and challenges that arise after a loss. These networks encompass family, friends, and professionals who offer different forms of support, each playing a unique role in the healing process. As the old saying goes, "It takes a village." In this case, it takes a village to support someone being impacted by grief because it affects each person differently.

Family Support

Family members are the closest and most immediate sources of support during times of grief. They share a deep connection and understanding of the deceased and the dynamics of the family unit. Family support can involve emotional support, shared reminiscing, and the opportunity to grieve together. Family members can provide a safe space to express emotions openly and without judgment, offering a sense of belonging and comfort. They can also collaborate in making practical arrangements, organizing funeral or memorial services, and addressing legal or financial matters.

Friends and Peers

Friends, close acquaintances, and peers can provide invaluable support during the grieving process. They offer companionship, a listening ear, and a non-judgmental space for sharing thoughts and feelings. Friends may not have the same familial ties, but they can offer a different perspective and provide a sense of normalcy and distraction through social activities or simply being present. Friends and peers who have experienced similar losses can offer empathy and relate to the grief journey, creating a sense of solidarity and understanding. It is important to have someone other than a family member to talk to or depend on during the grieving process.

Professional Support

Grief can be a complex and overwhelming experience, and professional support is crucial in helping individuals navigate their emotions and find healing. Grief counselors, therapists, psychologists, or social workers specialize in providing support and guidance through the grieving process. They offer a safe and confidential space to explore emotions, develop coping strategies, and work through the challenges unique to each individual's grief journey. Professionals can provide validation, help identify healthy ways of coping, and offer tools for self-care and resilience. Often times in a school setting, if someone passes away all of sudden whether it's a faculty member or student, grief counselors are on hand to help students or staff manage their loss.

Support Groups

Support groups bring together individuals who have experienced similar losses, creating a community where participants can share their stories, emotions, and challenges. Support groups offer a unique environment where individuals can feel understood and accepted. They provide opportunities for companionship, validation, and learning from others who are on a similar journey. Support groups are often facilitated by professionals or volunteers with expertise in grief, ensuring a safe and supportive space for participants.

The role of support networks is not limited to offering emotional support. They can also assist in practical matters, such as providing meals, running errands, or helping with childcare. Support networks can serve as a valuable resource for information, referrals, and assistance in navigating complex legal, financial, or logistical matters that may arise after a loss.

It is important to remember that support networks can evolve and change over time. Some relationships may strengthen, while others may fade. What matters most is finding a network that provides comfort, understanding, and validation during the grieving process. The combination of family, friends, and professionals offers a comprehensive support system that can help individuals find solace, resilience, and hope as they navigate the challenging terrain of grief.

Chapter 4: How to Heal through Grief

I really don't think there is a true way to heal from grief. I think there are some things that you can do to help deal with it. I am continuing with my online college classes and work full time. I have to keep busy to keep my mind off of things. If I don't, I will constantly worry about them. I think about my mother all the time because I have a lot of pictures of her and then family pictures. One particular practice that I do once a month is getting my nails done. I am also continuing with my writing. In fact, this book is dedicated to my mother. I plan to write more books and expand the types of books I write. I will be able to take some personal life experiences and turn them into a book.

Section 1: Finding a meaning in loss

Finding meaning in loss can be a transformative and healing process. When we experience loss, it is natural to question the purpose and significance of our pain. However, within the depths of grief, there lies an opportunity to discover profound meaning and embark on a journey of healing. In this section, we will explore strategies and examples of how individuals can find meaning in their losses and navigate the path towards healing.

Reflect on Personal Growth

Loss can serve as a catalyst for personal growth and transformation. A person has to take time to reflect on how the loss has shaped them as an individual. Consider the lessons learned, the strengths that emerged, and the values that have been redefined. Ask yourself how you have grown or changed as a result of the loss and how you can use these insights to shape your future.

Example

After losing a loved one, a person may reflect on the importance of cherishing relationships and living in the present moment. This newfound awareness may inspire them to prioritize connection, express gratitude, and live a more purposeful life. I find that although I form relationships with people, I make sure that I don't get too close to anyone.

Seek Connections and Support

It is important to find meaning in losing my mother by connecting with others who have lost a parent. I have a close friend that I mentioned earlier that I can relate to. I have thought about support groups. A coworker mentioned that she joined a church group that dealt with grief to talk about her experience. My support group has helped me to become stronger through my time of grief.

Example

Having a close friend who have experienced a loss like mine makes a difference. She can make a connection like other people can't. Through sharing stories, supporting one another, and advocating for causes related to parent loss, individuals can find a sense of purpose and contribute to a community dedicated to raising awareness and supporting one another.

Engage in Acts of Remembrance

Honoring the memory of the person or thing that was lost can be a powerful way to find meaning. Create rituals, memorials, or traditions that allow you to celebrate their life and keep their memory alive. In order to honor or remember the person, someone could light a candle, plant a tree, write letters, or organize events that pay tribute to their legacy.

Examples

When I was in 8th grade, the middle school building burned down. It was a big loss to the students and to the community. It was an electrical fire. I remember waking up one morning to hear that we were not going to school that day because of an electrical fire. The student council had a tree ceremony and bought a plaque in memory of the building. Then when the counselor at my school passed away, the school had a memorial and I wrote a poem called "A Greenwave Angel" for the principal to read at the memorial service. Just recently when the secretary died, the school made a plaque in her honor that hangs by the front doors to celebrate her memory.

Find Purpose Through Service

Channeling grief into acts of service can bring profound meaning and fulfillment. Engage in volunteer work or charitable endeavors that align with the values and interests of the person or thing that was lost. By giving back to others, we can find solace in the knowledge that our pain has inspired positive change in the world.

Example

After experiencing the loss of a pet, someone may volunteer at an animal shelter, offering their time and care to homeless animals. By providing love and support to animals in need, they find healing and purpose while honoring the memory of their beloved companion.

Embrace Creative Expression

Engaging in creative outlets can be a powerful way to process grief and find meaning. Explore activities such as writing, painting, music, or dance to express your emotions and thoughts. Creative expression allows for catharsis, self-discovery, and the opportunity to share your experiences with others.

Example

A person who has lost a sibling may write a memoir or create a photo collage that captures their sibling's life and the impact they had on their own. By sharing their story, they find meaning in preserving their sibling's memory and helping others who may be navigating similar grief. This book is being written in my mother's honor.

Finding meaning in loss is a deeply personal and individual journey. It requires introspection, vulnerability, and a willingness to explore the depths of our emotions. Through reflection, connection, remembrance, service, and creativity, individuals can discover profound meaning, growth, and healing amidst their grief. It is through these acts that the transformative power of loss can be harnessed, leading to a renewed sense of purpose, hope, and resilience.

Section 2: Creating new narratives and identities post-loss

Honoring the memory of a loved one who has passed away is a beautiful and meaningful way to keep their spirit alive while finding solace and comfort in the midst of grief. It allows us to preserve their legacy, cherish the impact they had on our lives, and create a lasting connection with their memory. In this section, we will discuss various ways to honor a deceased loved one and begin the healing process.

Create a Memorial Space

I have a space in my living room that has photographs of my mother. I also have pictures on my computer. And I also have her jewelry that I wear.

Celebrate Milestones and Anniversaries

Each year during my mother's birthday, my brothers and I go to her gravesite to put new flowers at her gravestone. We also go and put new flowers for Valentine's Day, Mother's Day, and Christmas. It's our way of still honoring our mother. When she was here on earth, we would always celebrate those holidays with her. It brings me joy to look back on videos of the things that we did with her when she was alive. She was so happy. So now, I hope that she knows that we are carrying on her request to come back to the "home house" during holidays to celebrate her memory.

Carrying the Legacy

One of the best ways to honor the memory of a loved one who has passed on is to carry forward the values that they taught you. My mother loved to bake different goodies so I am getting into different things. One particular thing that she enjoyed doing was sewing. I plan to learn how to sew so I make different things like she did. I can definitely honor my mother's memory do things like that.

Share Their Story

I love talking about the different things my mother did in her lifetime. I am including in this book things my mother taught her children.

Performing Acts of Kindness

My mother believed in helping people so I continue to help people like she would. I also provide a listening ear for those who need to talk to someone.

Commemorate through Artistic Expression

The day after my mother's death, I wrote a poem in memory of her. I have also gathered up pictures of her and other family pictures that are close by to look at her face. A DVD was created for her funeral, but I plan to create something digital for my family to watch to continue having memories.

Remember through Rituals and Traditions

One of the biggest family traditions was for my mother to cook Sunday dinner. I am proud to say that I continue that tradition by cooking for the family every Sunday at my mother's house. In her lifetime, she told her children for every holiday and celebration to "come back to the home house" and that is what we have done. It makes me proud that we have been able to honor her request. It is even more satisfying that I am able to cook or bake some of the same things that she did. There is no cooking like mommy's, but I try my best to get close to it.

Honoring the spirit of my mother is my way of keeping her spirit alive and it gives me comfort in her absence. It is my testimony of love and the strong connection that I had to her. It is my way of still carrying on the tradition that she would do if she were still alive.

Honoring the spirit of my mother is my way of keeping her spirit alive and it give me comfort in her absence. It is my testimony of love and the strong connection that I had to her. It is my way of still carrying on the tradition that she would do if she was still alive.

Chapter 5: Special Circumstances

As stated earlier, grief hits everyone differently. As a teacher, I have had a couple of students who lost a parent at a very young age. As an adult, it is hard to lose a parent. So, as a child, I could not even imagine what they are going through. I remember taking food to a family during their time of grief. I also remember attending a funeral to support the family and being a school representative. Sometimes when a parent dies, a child will completely change their attitude. I have seen children shut down, withdrawn, and simply be confused about what happened. As a teacher, I could only be strong for them, be a source of grace, and be a rock for them if they needed someone to talk with.

Although it is difficult as a child to lose a parent, I feel it is difficult for an adult as well. I think it is difficult to work in a place where you remember calling your mother when you had a break and when you had the opportunity, just come back home to see her on a teacher workday. Those memories hit me really hard at times, but I know that my mother would want me to remain strong.

Section 1: Children and grief

When children experience grief, it can be a difficult con-
cept for them to comprehend. It is very important to provide them the necessary support to understand their emotions and begin the healing process. It is important to acknowledge a child's feelings. Adults must create a safe and
supportive environment where children feel comfortable
talking to them. Children must know that they have open
lines of communication and that their feelings are valid.
Adults must be patience because children will have a wide
variety of emotions. They will express their emotions about
grief differently than adults. These emotions can include:
sadness, anger, confusion, and sometimes joy. You must use
a language that they can understand at their age when
talking about grief. The use of concrete language is important along with clear and appropriate answers. Avoid using
language that could confuse them.

In addition, it is important to provide stability and make
sure that children continue with the regular routines that
they are familiar with during grief. This would include

having the same mealtime and bedtime. Consistency is the key to normalcy in the pain of grief. Anytime a child has questions about grief, it is important to give age appropriate answers and use a language that they can understand. Allow children to express themselves in an appropriate way. If a child has trouble with communication, then let the child draw, paint, tell a story, or play. These are just a few ways that a child can express their emotions in a non-threatening way.

Furthermore, children need a strong support system that includes family, friends, and professionals to help them deal with grief. They should share their thoughts and feelings so that adults can provide them with comfort and guidance. Children support groups can help them feel a sense of belonging. They must also be given an opportunity to remember their loved one who passed away. It may be that the children talk about their memories, write letters, or participate in activities that will help them celebrate the person's life. Children can participate in a memorial event or plant a tree in a person's memory. Sometimes, a child's grief can be overwhelming and a professional has to step in. A grief counselor or therapists can provide specialized support and guidance to help a child with grief.

It is important to remember that every child's grief is unique. As an adult, it is important to be patient and understand a child's emotions. By providing safety and support, you can help a child navigate their emotions and begin the healing.

Section 2: Supporting from a distance

Grief has no boundaries, and sometimes we find ourselves separated from our grieving loved ones by physical distance. Whether due to geographical constraints, travel limitations, or other circumstances, supporting someone through their grief from afar presents unique challenges. However, with empathy, and the power of technology, we can still provide meaningful support and foster connection during their time of loss. In this section, we will explore strategies for supporting grieving loved ones from a distance.

Maintain Regular Communication

Regular communication is crucial when supporting someone from a distance. You have to reach out to your loved one through phone calls, video chats, text messages, or emails. People have to know you are there for them and available to listen whenever they need to talk. Actively check in with them, expressing your genuine care and concern. Remember to be patient, as grief can fluctuate, and they may need different levels of support at different times.

Practice Active Listening

If your loved one opens up about their grief, be an attentive and compassionate listener. Allow them to express their emotions, thoughts, and memories without judgment or interruption. Provide a space for them to share their pain and validate their experiences. Ask open-ended questions to encourage them to delve deeper into their feelings and actively engage in the conversation.

Offer Emotional Support

Emotional support plays a vital role in helping someone cope with grief. Express your empathy and understanding, acknowledging the depth of their pain. Let me know it is okay to feel a range of emotions that you are there to support them through it all. Offer words of comfort, reassurance, and encouragement. Remind them that they are not alone in their grief and that you are standing by their side, even from a distance.

Send Thoughtful Reminders

Even when physically apart, you can still send tangible reminders of your love and support. Consider mailing handwritten letters, care packages, or thoughtful gifts that symbolize your presence and understanding. These gestures can provide comfort and remind your loved one that they are in your thoughts and that their grief matters to you.

Coordinate Practical Support

Practical support can alleviate some of the burden that accompany grief. Offer assistance in organizing memorial services, handling paperwork, or managing daily responsibilities. You can help coordinate meals, arrange for cleaning services, or assist with any other tasks that may be overwhelming for your loved one. Additionally, you can help them access local resources or connect them with professionals who can provide support in their area.

Foster Virtual Connection

Technology is vital to use to foster virtual connection and support. You can schedule virtual gatherings or online memorial services where friends and family come together to honor the person who passed away. Facilitate video calls where your loved one can share stories, memories, or moments of reflection with others. Creating virtual spaces for connection can provide a sense of community and belonging.

Encourage Self-Care

Remind your loved one about the importance of self-care during the grieving process. Encourage them to engage in activities that bring them comfort and solace, such as journaling, exercise, meditation, or creative outlets. Provide recommendations for grief-related resources, such as books, articles, or online support groups, which can offer additional guidance and coping strategies.

Be Mindful of Cultural and Religious Practices

Respect and honor your loved one's cultural and religious practices related to grief. Familiarize yourself with their traditions, rituals, or customs, and find ways to support them within those frameworks. If appropriate and feasible, participate in virtual religious or cultural ceremonies or provide resources that align with their beliefs.

Supporting grieving loved ones from a distance requires flexibility, empathy, and creative approaches to connection.

Section 3: Grief in the workplace

Grief is an inevitable part of life, and its impact can extend beyond our personal lives and into the workplace. When an employee experiences the loss of a loved one or is going through a grieving process, it is essential for organizations to provide a supportive environment that acknowledges their pain and helps them navigate through this difficult time. In this section, we will explore strategies for handling grief in the workplace with compassion and understanding.

Establish an Open and Supportive Culture

Create a culture where employees feel comfortable expressing their emotions and seeking support during times of grief. Foster an environment of empathy and understanding, where colleagues can share their experiences without fear of judgment or stigma. Encourage open communication, and let employees know that their well-being is a priority.

Implement Bereavement Leave and Flexible Policies

Offer bereavement leave as part of your organization's policies. Allow employees time off to grieve and attend to practical matters associated with loss, such as funeral arrangements and family responsibilities. Additionally, consider implementing flexible work arrangements, such as remote work or adjusted schedules, to accommodate the unique needs of grieving employees.

During my time of grief, I took a couple of days off, but I found out later that I could have taken additional days off based on the work policy. I wanted to get back in a basic routine so I could get my mind off of things. It is important to know the policy about grief because when it happens to someone else, you will be familiar with how much time they are entitled to have off. It is also important if employees need to have any additional time off.

Communicate with Sensitivity and Compassion

When communicating with a grieving employee, other employees must approach the conversation with sensitivity and compassion. Offer condolences and express genuine concern for their well-being. Be understanding of their emotional state and any changes in their work performance or availability. It is important to provide reassurance that their grief is acknowledged and supported within the workplace. You must also know whether or not someone wants to be approached about the topic. When I went back to work, I wanted things to continue as "business as usual." It took me a while before I could talk about death without getting emotional or crying about it.

Provide Resources and Support

It is important to make resources available to employees to support them during their grieving process. This may include information on grief counseling services, employee assistance programs, or support groups. Some companies need to consider organizing workshops or training sessions to educate employees and managers about grief and its impact on the workplace. Providing access to relevant literature or online resources can also be beneficial.

Offer Employee Support Programs

Establish employee support programs or Employee Resource Groups (ERGs) specifically focused on grief and loss. These programs can create a safe space for employees to share their experiences, receive guidance, and connect with others who have gone through similar situations. Such initiatives foster a sense of community and understanding within the workplace.

Encourage Flexibility and Accommodations

Grief affects individuals differently, and it is important to offer flexibility and accommodations to employees as they navigate their grief journey. This may involve adjusting workloads, providing additional time for assignments, or temporarily reassigning tasks. By demonstrating flexibility and understanding, organizations can alleviate additional stressors for grieving employees. I would work my alloted amount of time and go home immediately after. I am a private person so if I was going to cry, I was going to wait until I got home.

Foster Peer Support and Connection

It is important to encourage colleagues to support one another during times of grief. Foster an atmosphere of empathy and encourage team members to check in on each other and offer support. This can be done through regular team meetings, virtual gatherings, or designated channels for sharing and supporting one another. Peer support can provide comfort and understanding, as colleagues are often best positioned to offer support due to their shared work experiences. Several people checked on me during the process phone calls, text messages, and just stopping by to show that they cared.

Train Managers in Grief Support

Managers and supervisors need to have training on how to support employees through the grieving process. They need to have the necessary skills to recognize signs of grief, engage in compassionate conversations, and offer appropriate support. Managers and supervisors play a crucial role in creating a supportive work environment and can be instrumental in facilitating the healing process for grieving employees.

Handling grief in the workplace requires empathy, compassion, and a commitment to support employees during their most vulnerable moments. By establishing an open and supportive culture, implementing bereavement policies, communicating with sensitivity, providing resources and support, offering employee support programs, encouraging flexibility, fostering peer support and connection, and training managers in grief support, organizations can create an environment that acknowledges and nurtures the healing process for grieving employees.

Chapter 6: Conclusion

I must be honest. I have never read a book on grief, but I was compelled to write one. I am a firm believer that you really don't understand something until it happens to you. Many people can come up to you and say, "I'm sorry for your loss. My thoughts and prayers are with your family." My argument is that until you have had an experience of someone you are close to leave you and you know they will never return back to Earth, you don't understand. For my closest friends who have experienced what I have, I will talk to them more because they understand exactly what I am going through. Now, I can understand exactly how my mother felt and the grieving that she did over her mother. I would hug her and hate to see her cry, but she told me that one day I would understand what she was going through, and I can say now I do.

Section 1: How to embrace the journey of grief

I must say that grief over the loss of my mother is the toughest journey that I have had to go on. Grief has a traumatic effect when it involves the loss of a loved one. Even in the midst of grief, there is an opportunity for growth, healing, and a renewed sense of self. In this section, we will examine ways to manage grief with courage and resilience. Grief is a deeply personal and transformative journey that accompanies the loss of a loved one. It is a complex and multi-faceted experience that can be overwhelming and challenging. However, within the depths of grief lies an opportunity for growth, healing, and a renewed sense of self. In this section, we will examine ways to manage grief with courage and resilience.

Acknowledge and Accept Your Feelings

The first step in embracing the journey of grief is to acknowledge and accept the wide range of emotions that arise. Allow yourself to feel the pain, sadness, anger, confusion, and any other emotions that surface. One must understand that these feelings are a natural response to loss and are an essential part of the healing process. Embracing your emotions with compassion and without judgment will help you move forward in your journey.

Practice Self-Compassion and Self-Care

Self-compassion is crucial during the grieving process. It is important to be gentle and kind to yourself as you navigate through the ups and downs of grief. Allow yourself the time and space to heal at your own pace. Engage in self-care activities that nourish your mind, body, and soul. This may include spending time in nature, engaging in creative outlets, practicing mindfulness or meditation, seeking therapy or counseling, or simply giving yourself permission to rest and recharge. One activity that I participate in every month is getting my nails done. It is my new norm of receiving my own self-care.

Seek Support and Connection

You can't go through the emotions of grief alone. It's important to reach out to your support network, whether it be family, friends, support groups, or professional counselors. Share your thoughts, feelings, and experiences with trusted individuals who can provide a listening ear, empathy, and understanding. Connecting with others who have experienced similar losses can be particularly valuable, as it creates a sense of belonging and validation. I have had a good connection with friends who have been through the same ordeal that I have. We are able to support each other.

Cultivate Resilience and Adaptability

Grief can be a transformative experience that challenges our sense of self and our worldview. Embracing the journey of grief involves cultivating resilience and adaptability in the face of adversity. The path of healing is not linear and there will be setbacks along the way. I am using this experience to embrace the opportunity to grow, learn, and adapt to the changes that loss brings. I plan to cultivate resilience by focusing on my strengths, practicing positive coping strategies, and seeking meaning and purpose in my life.

Explore Grief Rituals and Practices

Engaging in grief rituals and practices can provide a sense of structure and meaning during the grieving process. These rituals can be personal and tailored to your beliefs and preferences. I currently have a memorial space where I write in a journal to honor my mother. These practices can help you express your emotions, connect with your inner self, and find solace in the midst of grief.

Find Meaning and Purpose

Embracing the journey of grief involves seeking meaning and purpose in the face of loss. I can reflect on the different values that my mother taught me and I still live by those same values today. Consider ways to honor the memory of your loved one through acts of kindness, volunteering, or engaging in activities that were meaningful to them. Finding purpose amidst grief can bring a sense of fulfillment and contribute to your healing process.

Embrace Growth and Transformation

Grief has the potential to transform us in profound ways. Embrace the growth that comes from navigating through loss. You must allow yourself to evolve, develop a deeper understanding of life's complexities, and cultivate a greater appreciation for the present moment. Embracing the journey of grief involves embracing your own personal growth and the possibility of finding a new version of yourself as you move forward.

Section 2: Moving forward with hope and resilience

It is important to allow yourself to grieve as a part of the healing process. The first step is to give yourself permission to feel and express all of the emotions that come with grief. You can't deny these emotions because it is a part of the healing process. Denying these emotions will make it more difficult for peace and acceptance.

By allowing yourself to grieve, you are acknowledging the pain. You must give yourself some time and space to experience these emotions without any type of guilt. These are natural feelings because of loss. If you allow yourself to grieve, then you have a better opportunity to heal. You have to understand and process your emotions in order to get peace and acceptance. It's fine to cry, scream, or just be quiet. Two things that have always helped me have been to write in a journal and talk to a good friend. These are ways to move forward in healing and hope.

Talking to someone you trust can be a powerful tool in navigating the journey of grief. When you are grieving, it is essential to find a safe and supportive space where you can openly express your thoughts and emotions. Sharing your grief with someone you trust allows you to release pent-up feelings, gain perspective, and find comfort in knowing that you are not alone in your experience.

Choosing the right person to confide in is crucial. Look for someone who is compassionate, nonjudgmental, and willing to listen without offering unsolicited advice. This could be a close friend, family member, therapist, or support group. Trusting someone with your grief means finding someone who can hold space for your pain, validate your emotions, and provide a compassionate ear.

When talking to someone you trust about your grief, it is important to be honest and vulnerable. Allow yourself to share your deepest feelings, fears, and memories associated with your loss. Opening up about your grief can be difficult, but it can also bring a sense of relief and validation as you release your emotions and thoughts.

By talking to someone you trust, you can gain new insights and perspectives on your grief. Your trusted confidant may offer comforting words, share their own experiences, or provide guidance on coping strategies. Sometimes, simply having someone listen attentively can be incredibly healing and validating.

Remember that talking about your grief is not a one-time conversation. Grief is a process that unfolds over time, and your emotions may fluctuate. Regularly check in with your trusted person and continue to share your journey. As you do so, you will find that talking about your grief with someone you trust can bring immense comfort, support, and a renewed sense of hope as you navigate the path of healing.

It is better when you have someone to talk to that has been through the same experience as you have. When I talk to people about grief, I talk to the ones who know what I am going through. People can offer their sympathy and condolences, but until you experience, you really don't understand it.

Remembering that you are not alone in your grief can provide solace and comfort during the challenging times. Grief can often make you feel isolated, as if no one else understands your pain. However, the truth is that many people have experienced profound loss and understand the depths of sorrow that grief brings.

Grief is a universal human experience. From ancient times to the present, people from all walks of life have faced loss and grappled with the emotions that accompany it. Recognizing this shared experience reminds you that your feelings are valid, normal, and part of the human condition.

Section 3: Resources for continued support

In the journey of grief, it is essential to know that there are various resources available to help you cope with your loss. These resources can provide support, guidance, and solace during this challenging time. Here are some valuable resources to consider:

Grief Support Groups

Joining a grief support group can offer a safe and understanding environment to share your experiences, emotions, and challenges with others who have also experienced loss. These groups often provide a sense of community, validation, and an opportunity to learn from others who are on a similar journey.

Counseling and Therapy

Professional counseling and therapy can be instrumental in helping you navigate the complexities of grief. A therapist specializing in grief counseling can provide a confidential space for you to explore your emotions, develop coping strategies, and find healthy ways to process your grief. They can offer guidance and tools tailored to your unique needs.

Books and Literature

There is a wealth of literature available that addresses grief and offers insights and support. Reading books written by grief experts or individuals who have experienced loss can provide comfort, validation, and practical advice. These resources can help you gain a deeper understanding of grief and discover coping mechanisms that resonate with you.

Online Communities and Forums

The internet offers a wide range of online communities and forums where individuals experiencing grief can connect, share their stories, and provide support to one another. Participating in these virtual spaces can help you feel less alone, access a diverse range of perspectives, and find solace in the understanding and compassion of others.

Retreats and Workshops:

Grief retreats and workshops provide immersive and focused environments for healing and self-reflection. These programs often incorporate therapeutic techniques, group activities, and individual reflection to facilitate healing and personal growth. Attending such events can offer a dedicated space to process your grief and gain valuable tools for navigating your journey.

Religious and Spiritual Support

If you have a religious or spiritual inclination, seeking support from your faith community or spiritual leaders can be beneficial. Many religious organizations offer grief counseling, support groups, rituals, and ceremonies that can provide a sense of comfort, meaning, and connection during your grieving process.

Remember, each person's journey of grief is unique, and the resources that resonate with you may differ from others. Explore these options, and don't hesitate to reach out for support. The availability of these resources ensures that you don't have to face your grief alone. Utilize these tools to find solace, healing, and a path towards embracing life with renewed hope and resilience.

Acknowledgements

I would like to express my deepest gratitude to the spirit of my late mother, Mrs. Alma Rhodes. Her unwavering love, strength, and courage continue to inspire me every day. This book, <u>Handling Grief: A Guide to Understanding and Coping with Loss</u>, stands as a testimony to her enduring spirit and the profound impact that my mother had on my life.

To my dear mother, thank you for being that shining light in my journey. All the love and support that you provided me gave me the strength to manage this challenging endeavor. Even though you are no longer physically with us, your presences and wisdom will resonate through these pages, and will offer solace and comfort to those who are managing the painful terrain of grief.

I would also like to acknowledge the invaluable support and encouragement that came from my brothers and friends. Your strong belief in me and your willingness to lend an ear during the tears, strong emotions, doubt, fear, and pain have been instrumental in bringing this book to publication. I am truly blessed to have such a wonderful and remarkable support system.

I am indebted to the various individuals who have shared their personal stories of grief and loss. Your courage in opening up about your experiences has enriched this book and made it a reflection of the diverse paths we walk through in grief. The resilience in others has been true inspiration.

Finally, I would like to say thank you to my readers. It is my hope that the words on these pages will offer you solace, guidance, and a glimmer of hope during the darkest times of your life. May you find the comfort in knowing that you are truly not along in your journey of grief.

In memory of my beloved mother, Mrs. Alma Rhodes, I dedicate this book. Your love continues to guide me, and your legacy lives on through these pages. Though the pain of losing you will always be present, I am forever grateful for the strength and courage that you instilled in me. Your spirit will forever and always be cherished.

About the Author

Dr. Ann B. Rhodes is the author of <u>From the Beginning Until Now</u>, her first book of poetry, which went into publication in 2016. When she was an elementary school student, God blessed her with a talent that she didn't discover until she was in sixth grade, during her middle school years. Over several years, a variety of her poems have been published in the *Hogansville Herald*, *LaGrange Daily News*, and even WSB-TV in a "Please, Stop the Violence" campaign. Three poems, "A Great Man," The Greatest Easter Gift," and "What is a Mother? have been published in different poetry anthologies throughout the United States. The poem <u>A Great Man</u> is a part of a CD collection incorporated by Poetry.com. Dr. Rhodes has published poetry books, devotional books, and children's books. She is currently an elementary school teacher with a doctoral degree. She enjoys writing poetry and spreading God's message to people all over the world.

***

Did you know... Reader reviews are very important to self-published and Indie authors. We fuel our success and growth and help other readers find our work. If you loved this book, scan the QR code to leave a review filled with stars. It will help me out.

Handling Grief QR Code

***

Don't forget your gift, scan the QR to tell me where to send
it.

www.ingramcontent.com/pod-product-compliance
Lightning Source LLC
Chambersburg PA
CBHW060622200326
41521CB00007B/861